What To Do When
Overeating Gets Out of Hand

Stop Overeating By Conquering Emotions

By: Octavia Black

TABLE OF CONTENTS

Octavia Black

PUBLISHERS NOTES

Disclaimer

DEDICATION

This book is dedicated to individuals like my uncle Roy who struggle to beat overeating every day.

Octavia Black

CHAPTER 1- WHAT IS OVEREATING AND WHAT ARE THE ROOT CAUSES?

When people hear the words eating disorder, most only think of disorders in which one is starving in an effort to lose weight. While starving oneself is in fact an eating disorder, there is another eating issue that millions of people struggle with and that is overeating.

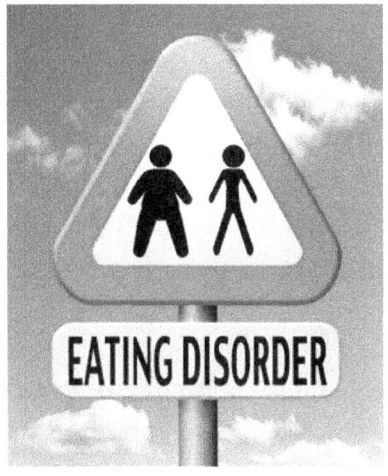

Overeating is known to occur when a person consumes an excessive amount of food at one time. Sure this is something that most of us have done at one time or another. Perhaps, at a family get together, a major holiday, or at a buffet and that once every now and then overeating binge is normally not extremely harmful to health. Instead, it is when an individual chooses to compulsively overeat several times throughout a week or over a time period that issues start to develop. If someone is sitting down several times a week and finishing off a bag of chips, several pizzas, or an entire gallon of ice cream by themselves, then they are compulsively overeating at a level that their health may start to suffer from.

If someone is in fact overeating on a pretty regular basis, then normally the cause isn't just because they are at a buffet or a family get-together, but actually because of a root cause that make them feel like they have the need to constantly feel hungry or need to be eating large quantities. The first root cause that will cause many people to overeat is actually a simple one to correct and that is overeating and binging due to boredom.

If someone is bored and has nothing exciting to do, then they may find that they have emptied an entire bag of chips by themselves while just lounging around the house. Boredom is one of the easier causes of overeating to correct. Basically if that is the cause of overeating, then that person can just make a few lifestyle adjustments that get them up and moving and find an activity that fills their down time to keep that food out of their hands.

There are several deeper root causes of overeating that aren't quite as easy to address as binging because of boredom. These causes are normally due to an individuals' emotional health and often take years of counseling and therapy to address and overcome.

Eating because of an emotional or mental health issues is often the result of poor coping strategies in place or deeper rooted issues from childhood that cause someone to overeat. When it comes to poor coping mechanisms, basically someone doesn't know how to handle stress or anxiety in their life, because they never learned how to appropriately handle everyday stressors in life or larger life events and the only thing they know to do to cope with such stress is to turn to food.

Octavia Black

If this is the reason for overeating, then trying to eliminate as much stress as possible from the person's life may be a possible fix; however, due to reality this is not always entirely possible. In addition to trying to eliminate the stress and anxiety, then the person can also learn ways to release and deal with their anxiety in positive ways, such as journaling or exercising and in some cases may wish to seek medical treatment and medicine to help relieve their stress and anxiety.

Besides anxiety and stress causing overeating, perhaps the hardest cause of overeating to treat is when someone is overeating because of habits and issues that were developed during childhood. Unfortunately, many parents never try to figure out what their child is really asking for when they are crying as infants or toddlers and instead of trying to successfully meet their child's needs, they instead just assume the child is hungry and stuff its mouth with a bottle or with food. This can then cause issues of overeating as an adult.

What is taught at an early age by such parenting techniques of feeding for comfort instead of other methods to comfort, teaches someone at an early age that you eat when you need comforted. So when this person reaches adulthood, that line of thinking is still there. If you have had a bad day at work, then you eat as much as you want until your day goes away. Going through a divorce and need comfort, then why not eat a gallon of ice cream by yourself, is how the thought process works. This cycle is extremely hard to break, as this is how you were taught to eat when growing up; however, it isn't an impossible thing to take control of.

While the biggest consequence of overeating and not dealing with the root causes to stop the issue is obesity, the fact is that there are many other health related issues that may occur as a result of overeating. If a person is overeating a specific food group on a regular basis, then that it itself will increase health risks. For example, if it is sweets that someone is eating on a binge, then they will be more prone to developing diabetes. If the choice of someone who binges is normally high in fat and cholesterol, then they will be more likely to develop heart diseases and heart problems.

Besides physical consequences and the damage to ones' body, there are also other aspects of overeating to consider. Once someone binges enough to cause weight gain, then they become limited to what sports and recreational activities they can participate in, which leads to more weight gain and then in turn to more emotional problems. Also, keep in mind that if someone is binging while at work that their work performance may be affected, which in turn could have a financial impact should one lose their job because of their binge eating.

If you are a binge eater or someone you know fits the characteristics of what an overeater is, then it is strongly advised that treatment be sought. Taking the first step will be hard, but that step must be taken to stop the cycle of overeating and to take one's health back.

Chapter 2- What is Emotional Eating?

Satisfying hunger is not the only reason some people eat. Food is often used as a reward, a stress reliever, or a source of comfort. Emotional problems are not solved with emotional eating. Often eating emotionally makes a person feel worse than before. The emotional issue is not solved. Guilt from overeating sets in. Recognizing the triggers that cause emotional eating is essential to getting the habit under control.

Making room for dessert when you already feel full and diving into ice cream when depressed are all forms of emotional eating. Eating is an attempt to fill an emotional need. Occasional rewards or pick me ups are not necessarily bad. If eating is the usual coping mechanism when bored, tired, stressed, lonely, angry, or upset, an unhealthy cycle has developed. This needs to be addressed.

Eating only feels good for a moment. The impulse that triggers the cycle does not fill the emotional hunger. Unnecessary calories consumed add to the emotional distress. Blame for overeating and lack of willpower occurs. Learning healthy ways to cope are eliminated. It becomes more difficult to control weight. People in this cycle feel powerless against emotions and foods.

Emotional eaters eat more when feeling stressed. Eating takes place even when hunger is not present. Eating until a person feels stuffed becomes part of the daily routine. Emotional eating is an attempt to feel better. Food becomes like a friend. A false sense of safety is felt. Feeling out of control around food happens.

What To Do When Overeating Gets Out of Hand

Emotional hunger is very powerful. It can be mistaken for physical hunger. Knowing the difference is important in breaking the cycle. There are clues to look for that aid in differentiating them.

Emotional hunger comes on instantly. There is an overwhelming sense of urgency. Unless a long time has elapsed since eating, physical hunger gradually presents itself.

Craving specific foods is indicative of emotional hunger. Sugary snacks or fatty foods provide a rush of sorts. When someone is truly hungry, almost anything will cure the hunger, healthy foods included.

Without realizing what is happening, an emotional eater can devour an entire package of chips or a container of ice cream. Being full does not satisfy emotional hunger. Eating to satisfy physical hunger is done with awareness of the action. The eater is satisfied when full.

Emotional hunger is not identified by a growling stomach or pangs in the belly. Cravings that can seem to be impossible to erase from the mind occur. Specific smells, tastes or textures are needed to pacify.

Shame, guilt, and regret accompany emotional eating. The guilt is a sign that the eater knows that eating is not just for nourishment of the body. Emotional eaters feel bad about themselves.

There are different reasons for emotional eating. Understanding personal triggers helps put an end to the problem. Becoming aware of the feelings, places, and situations that cause emotional eaters to seek comfort from food is important.

Stress is part of nearly all health issues. A stress hormone, called cortisol, is released when the environment is fast-paced and chaotic.

This hormone causes cravings for foods high in fat, sugar, or salt. Looking for emotional comfort from food is proportional to the amount of stress present.

Shame, resentment, loneliness, anxiety, sadness, fear, and anger are uncomfortable emotions that emotional eaters try to silence or stuff down. It is an attempt to avoid the emotion. Some people eat for lack of something better to occupy their time. Food fills and an unfulfilled empty void. It distracts from feelings of dissatisfaction and purposelessness.

If parents rewarded an emotional eater with food when young, the emotionally-based habit can carry over to adulthood. Nostalgia can drive people to eat emotionally. Cherished memories like baking cookies with Grandma, family gatherings around a table of home cooked meals, or grilling with Dad can cause emotional eaters to search for some specific foods.

Attendance at social gatherings can be a problem. It seems as though everyone else is overindulging, so why not join the crowd. Food at these kinds of events is often left to enjoy during the duration of the party. This makes for easy access. Snacking occurs throughout the party.

Keeping a diary that tracks mood and food is one way to learn the specific causes of emotional eating. Anytime that overeating, or the compulsion to do so, occurs, make an entry in the diary. Record what was eaten or desired. Also pen what was upsetting and the feelings before, during, and after eating.

What To Do When Overeating Gets Out of Hand

A pattern will emerge. Being around critical people, being under deadlines, or attending family functions may be the sources of stress. Once identified, healthier ways to feed emotions can be sought.

Emotional fulfillment alternatives are needed. Calling someone, playing with a pet, or looking at cherished mementos may alleviate depression or loneliness. Dancing, squeezing a stress ball, or going for a brisk walk may relieve anxiety. A cup of tea, a bath, scented candles, or a warm blanket may drive away exhaustion. Reading, comedy, outdoor activities, or hobbies can prevent boredom.

Just because past endeavors to resist temptation have failed, does not mean the problem cannot be conquered. Emotional eating is nearly automatic and mindless; notice the nearly. Taking a pause and reflecting for just a moment before giving into a craving, gives the opportunity to make a better decision. Waiting for a minute or two allows the eater to check the need. Even if the decision to eat is made, there will be a better understanding of why it occurred. A different response may come next time.

Allowance of uncomfortable feelings can be scary. A fear of never ending pain or difficulty arises. Obsessing and suppressing emotions can be even more painful and difficult. Emotions subside quickly and lose power over one obsessing when they are allowed to be felt.

Emotions are a window to the soul. Being open emotionally helps to discover and understand deep fears and desires. Keys to frustration and things that cause happiness become apparent.

Healthy lifestyles include being strong physically, being rested, and being relaxed. Inevitable hiccups can be dealt with in a better way. Exercise and sleep play a part in a healthy lifestyle. Exercise reduces stress and boosts mood and energy levels. Sugary snacks are craved by the body for an energy boost. Eight hours of sleep helps reduce and control cravings.

CHAPTER 3- WHAT ARE CRAVINGS AND HOW DO THEY CONTRIBUTE TO OVEREATING?

A craving, by definition, is an intense desire for something. A craving for food usually has very little to do with hunger. When it comes to food, everyone has experienced a craving for something unhealthy at least once in his life. For many people who are on a restrictive diet, a craving can become tortuous, leaving the person on the diet feeling completely defeated as he can think of very little else besides fulfilling the craving.

There are many theories as to why humans experience food cravings. One theory suggests that when a person consumes sugar, the same area of the brain that produces addiction is activated. Hence, for some people, consuming sugary foods or simple carbohydrates, which later turn into sugar in the body, can become an addiction because that area that controls addiction is being triggered. Another theory suggests that sugars and carbohydrates produce endorphins in the brain when they are consumed.

These endorphins give the person a sense of relaxation and an overall sense of well-being. Another explanation as to why humans have food cravings lies in nutritional deficiencies. For example, if a person craves salt, he is probably dehydrated and needs to replenish his electrolyte count. It could also be a sign of stroke or diabetes, in some people. When a woman is on her menstrual cycle, she often complains about having a craving for chocolate. This is because chocolate contains the mineral iron and iron is lost during a woman's menstrual cycle. A craving for dairy products could indicate a deficiency in vitamin D. New research is showing that cravings result from a culmination of these theories, and not just from one particular cause.

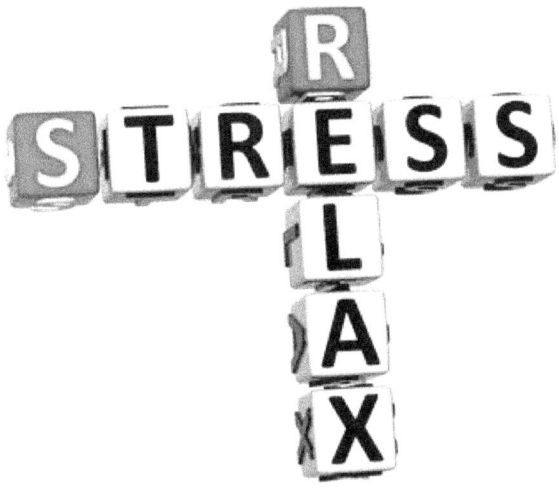

Unfortunately, not being able to control food cravings can result in overeating, thereby resulting in obesity. This can happen due to classical conditioning of the brain. People are so exhausted from work and carry a lot of stress with them. The human brain strives for a feeling of relaxation and well-being. Because of the "feel good" chemicals released to the brain when a person eats sugar or carbohydrates, the person associates these foods with feelings of well-being. He may not even be cognitively aware of the association, but his body and his brain are, and his brain will make sure that his body submits to the craving in an attempt to feel better.

Overeating can also be a result of the sugar and carbohydrates triggering the same responses in the brain that addiction does. Anyone who has struggled with addiction of any kind understands that the more a person consumes of the addiction, the more he is going to have to consume in order to achieve the same "high". Food cravings are no different than any other addiction. The more sugar and carbohydrates a person consumes, the more he will have to consume in order to achieve the same sense of well-being that previously came from a smaller amount of food. The brain becomes immune to the sugar previously consumed and needs more in order to release the same number of endorphins. Therefore, the person overeats in order to feel more relaxed.

The theory that suggests that overeating comes from a specific nutritional deficiency offers another explanation of why people who have cravings overeat. This theory suggests that when a person has a nutritional deficiency, he does not understand what his body is trying to tell him. Therefore, he misinterprets his body's signals and reaches for the wrong food.

For example, if he is dehydrated and needs water, he craves salt so that his body will hold onto the little amount of water he has in his body. Instead of recognizing his craving for salt as a desperate plea from his body to drink water, he instinctively reaches for a bag of salty potato chips. However, after consuming an entire bag of potato chips, he is still not satisfied. His lack of satiety comes from not understanding what his body was really asking him to do.

Understanding the reasons behind cravings can help a person who overeats regularly. By understanding the link between the brain and what a person craves can help him adjusts his behavior to ensure that he does not overeat. For example, if after a stressful day the individual is craving carbohydrates, it is probably because his brain is trying to restore balance and increase endorphins.

However, the individual can release those endorphins simply by exercising. By using exercise, instead of carbohydrates, to fulfill the brain's need to create balance and a sense of well-being, he can effectively control his impulse to overeat. If a woman is craving chocolate during her menstrual cycle, she can realize that she may have an iron deficiency caused by her cycle. By understanding her deficiency, she can replace dark green vegetables in her diet for chocolate. By satisfying her body's need for iron, she can reduce her craving for chocolate and, thereby, reduce the possibility of overeating.

Overeating has taken a toll on most of society's health. By eating too much of the wrong kinds of food, people end up consuming too many calories. There is an epidemic in society of individual's with heart disease, Type II diabetes, and other diet related illnesses. People are eating too much and exercising too little. Many diets fail because they restrict what the individual can eat. Many diets fail to educate the individual about cravings and why he craves certain foods. Because of this lack of information, many diets fail within a few weeks or a few months.

Fulfilling one's cravings is about self-preservation. The body and brain are designed to preserve themselves in a sense of well-being. However, in a world that demands so much from the individual, he can easily become extremely stressed very easily. The brain and body were just not designed for so much stress. In addition, the brain and body require certain nutrients in order to survive. However, getting the proper nutrition is difficult in a world that thrives on convenience foods. The question remains to be answered is if humans will continue to hurt their brain and bodies or help them.

CHAPTER 4- HOW TO DIAGNOSE THE EMOTIONAL EATER

The reasons why some people have what is considered eating and food related issues are vast. This is because there are some people who simply eat for the love of food and then there are others who have less control as they tend to eat based on emotions. This is why the need to better understand how to diagnose an emotional eater is high since eating disorders can develop based on emotional reasons that cause one to eat in a manner not conducive to good health or healthy eating.

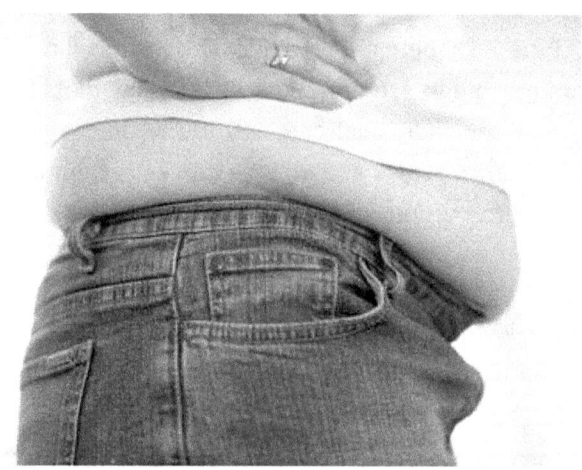

Emotional eating is one issue that can come about at just about any age and can also happen after a life changing event. It is something that can be hard to handle and manage alone and thus those who have such issues need to be assessed, evaluated and professionally determined to have an emotional eating issue so that things can be done to change those habits which can be bad for ones well being and overall health.

Emotional eaters tend to be those who have some deep down need to satisfy their feelings of loneliness, emptiness or even sadness. This is the predominant manner that triggers emotional eating and for many this is something that happens from time to time. In fact, it is actually common and acceptable for one to go through a relationship change or have a bad day and seek comfort in foods that make them feel better. Some people find the taste or even the smell of certain foods calming and this is a form of emotional eating that is fine if it only happens from time to time. The issue becomes one that is concerning when it impacts ones health and increases in frequency over time. Emotional eating, since it is rooted in the mental state of the person, is something that takes time to work through and eventually overcome.

The most common way to begin making a diagnosis of an emotional eater is to have that individual start keeping a food log or diary. This is an extremely helpful tool once the individual understands best how to keep the right notes about what they eat, when they eat and why they eat. It is a process that will take a few attempts to get right; however, once one starts logging all of their food and drink intake patterns begin to emerge rather quickly that can be highly beneficial in determining if the person is truly to be considered an emotional eater. This is the ideal starting point as it is partially the responsibility of the emotional eater to keep those records for professionals to use in their assessment.

Once this chronicling of eating habits has been going on for at least a few weeks or even a month or more one can then really sit down with the person and start to assess the situation in a more comprehensive manner. This is because the log or diary should be very detailed. This means that the person who is charting their eating habits needs to write down everything they consume each day, the time of day the food was eaten and also what they were doing before they ate. In addition, it is imperative that the person write down what their mood was before, during and after eating. This is key as it helps to showcase the thought process behind eating and this is what will be sued to further determine why one eats what and when they do on a regular basis.

The use of this highly detailed journal is then what is used by a trained professional to make that determination in regards to whether the person in fact does fall under the category of being an emotional eater. There are some emotional eaters that tend to become overweight or even obese if they have such emotional issues that they find comforted only through food.

The majority of these people have issues that extend far beyond food dependency and comfort; as some were punished with food as a child, deprived of food by others at some point in their life or even shamed in to thinking they ate too little or too much at points in their life. These are all the various types of issues that need explored by those who have the right training in the issues surrounding emotional eating and the challenges is poses to those who suffer through such an issue.

The extensive work that goes in to understanding and truly figuring out if one is an emotional eater needs to be done in stages and needs to involve a lot of two way communication between the professional handling the patient and the patient. This is because the truth and reasons behind the eating issues only come out when the talks are in depth and thus examine the root causes.

This is where that all important food journal becomes relevant as it serves a purpose in that it is useful as a guide to talking through the issue. This is because when charted correctly that log shows both patient and professional the thoughts that were being felt when food was consumed. This is the point where a treatment or therapeutic plan can be orchestrated to help combat those emotional eating habits.

Emotional eaters act the way they do, in regards to satisfying a need through the use of food, because they have not been taught nor conditioned to handle those emotions in more productive or healthier ways. This is why the need is great for one who even suspects that they have an issue with food that is centered on how they feel as it can become highly problematic over time and thus cause a situation that becomes a habit which gets harder and harder to break as time passes. In fact, once a person knows they eat based on emotions they can work towards finding alternate means to express their feelings, stave off thoughts that prompt eating and eventually learn to have a better relationship with both food and themselves.

CHAPTER 5- HOW TO TREAT EMOTIONAL EATING

Treating overeating can be difficult because most people have been overeating for their entire lives. In our society where food is in abundance, it can be difficult to nip this harmful habit so that it does not spiral out of control. Being able to treat overeating can help you to lose weight and feel better, and it might also be able to help you save money on food. There are quite a number of techniques you can and should use if you would like to stop overeating and get your eating habits back into a more normal schedule.

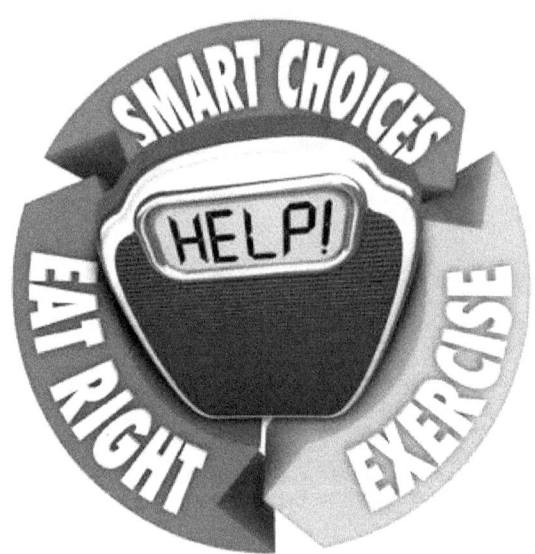

Portion Your Food

One of the best things you can do is to portion out your food when it comes to what you will be eating. Nowadays, a lot of snacks come in large value size bags that may leave you eating more in the end. The best thing for you to do would be to look at the label of the food you're eating and look at the serving size. For instance, a bag of chips might have about 30 chips for around 200 calories. When you open the bag, it can be very easy for you to eat 60 or 80 chips in one sitting simply because you are not paying attention.

The best way to portion out your food is to do so by looking at the suggested serving size on the food's label. Those 30 chips for 200 calories can be divided into bags. If you do not want to put chips in a re-sealable bag, you can always pour the chips into a small bowl. This will immediately force you to eat less simply because you do not have the bag right there in front of you at all times. This is one way that you will be able to avoid overeating and start kicking this habit.

Buy Pre-Portioned Foods

Another wonderful thing that you should think about buying would be pre-portioned foods and snacks. You can buy these in basically any supermarket. Just look for snacks that come in smaller individual bags and you will be able to simply grab and go without putting any thought into it. A lot of people have had success with these pre-portioned calorie pack snacks because it allows them to eat their favorite foods without necessarily sitting and measuring everything out.

One of the main issues with pre-portioned snacks and foods is that they do tend to be more expensive because the portioning work has already been done for you. Just look at a bag of your favorite cookies and compare them to the pre-portioned calorie packs on the store's shelf. You might notice that you get fewer cookies in the pre-portioned bag and it actually costs more. This might be a good idea for people who do not have a lot of time to portion out their foods, but it can become expensive if you have a tendency to buy a lot of these types of items.

Eat Less but More Often

Another way to treat overeating is to eat less food, but more often. For instance, you might be used to having a huge breakfast with an omelet and some toast with fruit or juice. Instead of having huge amounts of food all in one sitting, think about eating slightly less, but eat another small meal or snack in about two hours from your previous meal. This will keep you satisfied throughout the day and will avoid having you feel as though you are on a diet. No one wants to have the feeling of deprivation, so it might be good to eat small snacks and meals throughout the day.

Schedule Snacks and Meals

Another tip for treating overeating is to schedule out the specific meals and snacks you'll have in your day. Don't just go with the flow when you know you have issues with overeating because this can turn into a nightmare if you are not too careful. Know what you're going to eat and when you're going to eat it so that you know how many calories you'll be consuming in a day and you can avoid overeating. While this may seem strange at first for you, this can do wonders for you when it comes to kicking the bad habit of overeating.

Choose Lower Calorie Foods

Overeating is a habit that most people develop throughout the years and because of this, it is difficult to get rid of the habit fully or quickly.

One of the easiest ways to prevent weight gain from overeating is by simply choosing lower calorie foods instead of full-calorie ones on the local store shelf. For instance, you might love soda and drink it constantly, but you may not realize that you are consuming thousands of calories just in soda alone if you drink a lot of it. By switching to the diet variety or sugar-free variety of soda, you will be cutting hundreds and possibly thousands of calories from your diet each day.

The same theory can be applied to the types of foods that you eat. Let's say you are a big chip lover and enjoy nothing more than potato chips. Instead of the regular variety, consider switching to baked or a different brand that has less trans-fat. This will help to cut calories even if you're used to eating the entire bag.

By making these small changes to your daily lifestyle, you should be able to quickly and easily get over your habit of overeating and begin losing weight. This will benefit your health, mental well-being and even your wallet because you are not buying as much food for yourself. You will find that many of these tips become habitual for you so that they are easy to stick with over time and actually become more regular for you than your overeating was for your entire life. Overeating can be harmful in many ways, but there are tips to stop this habit.

CHAPTER 6- THE BENEFIT OF SUPPORT GROUPS FOR THE EMOTIONAL EATER

Emotional eating can be an extremely difficult problem that affects the lives of many people. Unlike other addictions where the substance can be avoided entirely, eating addictions have to be managed carefully because people cannot fully avoid food each day. There are some great things that someone can begin doing now that can give them the tools to overcome emotional eating. The right support groups can be very helpful in setting new patterns in life. This can give you insider information about others that are struggling, and you will also be able to meet those that have overcome this troubling problem.

One of the benefits of a support group for emotional eating is that you will learn new tools to combat this type of eating. Learning how to manage your stress better can be very helpful in overcoming emotional eating. Most people have a great deal of stress in their lives that is not managed properly. This can turn into a situation where eating is the outlet. There are many different ways that a person can manage stress that does not affect the diet. This can allow someone to not let stress affect the way they treat food.

Support groups can also put you in touch with people that are dealing with the exact same problem that you are. This can provide you with more tools than any other source. You will be exposed to people in all phases of recovery from food addiction. You may find answers to help you that you have not heard of before. This can give you a new perspective on how to overcome emotional eating, and these may be techniques that you use for life. People that are struggling with the same challenges as you are can be very welcoming when you first join this support group, and this can encourage you to attend more meetings.

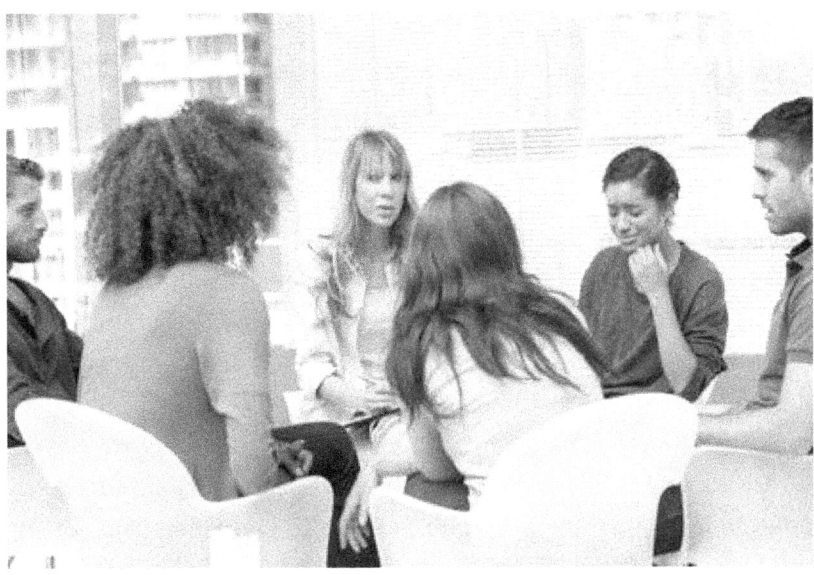

When you are around other people that suffer from emotional eating you will find that they come from all walks, and backgrounds. This can allow someone to feel more comfortable when they are in this group setting. Many people build friends very quickly in this type of setting. This is what a support group is all about. As you begin to feel more comfortable in this setting and with the people around you, it can allow you to really open up and get the most out of this supportive setting. The first time you visit this group can be very intimidating. Many support groups have a very relaxed setting allowing you to feel as comfortable as possible.

It can be very common to hide from your emotional eating. This may be a problem where you feel very alone, and you may not want others to know about the emotional eating you have been experiencing. Support groups are completely anonymous. This will allow you to attend this group, and no one in your life has to know unless you disclose this information to them. This is not a group that often meets in a public place, and you will find the discreetness you are looking for if this is important to your needs. You can tackle this problem without involving anyone in your life, and this is not something you will have to be ashamed about once you begin finding solutions to emotional eating problems.

Empowerment can be a huge factor when it comes to overcoming emotional eating. Many people feel powerless and stuck in this pattern. You may have certain triggers or times when you are most vulnerable to reckless eating habits. Recognizing your weaknesses can allow you to become extremely empowered. This can help you to have more control over something that made you feel out of control. It can be very important to understand what your specific triggers are when it comes to food. This support group can help you to understand not only how to overcome emotional eating, but also how to gain good eating habits for life.

There are a couple of different ways that you can attend a support group for emotional eating. You can find a physical location where you live. This will often be a meeting that you have to attend once per week, or less. This is something that you will find at your local community center in many cities. You can also choose to attend support groups online. This will put you in touch with people that are suffering from the same problem all over the United States. This can be a great support group for someone that is unable to travel to a physical location. You can still get some great benefits by reaching out to others online. You should make sure that you are choosing a group that is going to make you feel the most comfortable.

Changing you ways and learning new habits can be one of the biggest benefits of using a support group. Many people need to adjust eating habits, and there are some tools that can be gained from a support group that can be useful in helping you reach your goal. You may find with the right support you can finally lose weight and change your habits. This can make you happier and healthier as you begin to find new ways to manage stress and emotions better. You will learn to turn away from food, and these are lessons that can be invaluable if you have been unable to do this on your own.

The benefits of support groups for the emotional eater can be numerous. The biggest benefit is you can finally become the person you are meant to be. Eating will not control you any longer, and this can allow you to make better choices in your eating habits, and you will also learn tools to manage the triggers that lead you to emotional eating in the first place. Taking the first step in seeking out a support group can help you to be more motivated to make the changes that can really improve your life.

CHAPTER 7- OVEREATING: HOW TO PREVENT A RELAPSE

The diet industry is a multi-million dollar business fueled by people who are desperate to lose weight to become healthier and look better. However, even with all of the resources available only a small percentage of people are able to keep off the weight that was lost. Most of the time there is more weight gain after reaching the goal and ending the diet. This leads to frustration and the temptation to give up. While each person is unique as to why overeating is an issue, the following tips will assist those attempting to prevent a relapse.

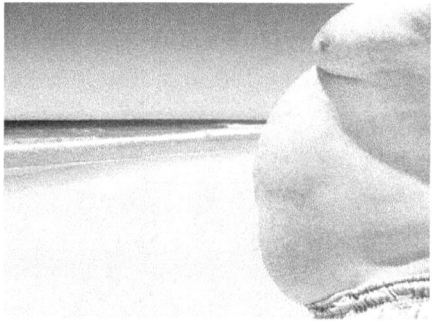

Dieters see their favorite foods daily. The smell, taste, and textures of favorite foods are unavoidable. Unlike other habits that rely on the offending temptation being "banished", dieters must face seemingly insurmountable odds to lose weight because every day they encounter the very thing that is contributing to their health issues. Office parties, holidays, dinners out, and movie theater concessions all contribute to overeating. Eating is not only a necessity it is social. People celebrate with food.

When it comes to diet, planning is everything. To prevent overeating, planned meals and snacks are the first line of defense. Successful dieters keep a meal log. This assists in preventing emotional or impulsive eating. If enjoying a dinner out, looking at the restaurant menu and choosing what foods to eat before arriving will help to prevent the temptation to overeat. Eating a good meal before going to the movies or attending the office party will keep the hors d'oeuvre table less interesting.

Enjoying regularly scheduled breakfast, lunch, and dinner without distraction is a way to indulge in the pleasure of eating. Eating slowly and savoring each bite gives the stomach time to tell the brain it is satisfied. Those who are overweight often eat too fast for the stomach to signal the brain that it is full, allowing consumption of more calories than necessary.

Avoiding television, technology, and work during mealtimes will allow the mind to recognize that it has eaten. When participating in activities at the same time as a meal, it is easy to view mealtime as an all-day event. Select specific areas to eat regular meals. This will signal the brain that these areas are for meals and it is inappropriate to eat elsewhere. This cuts down on the sometimes mindless grazing that is one of the culprits of weight gain.

Many people will taste test foods while cooking. This is a great way to add excess calories to the diet without realizing it because even after tasting the food, most will sit down and eat full servings. It is best to season the food to taste after serving.

When attempting to avoid overeating it is important to understand that meals do not have to be finished. It takes the brain about 20 minutes to receive the signal from the stomach that it is full. A person eating slowly may not feel the need to complete a full serving. Many dieters believe that it is shameful to waste food. Extra food may be shared with a friend or eaten as lunch the next day.

An optical illusion can prevent overeating. Using smaller plates trick the eye into believing that there is more food to eat than there actually is on the plate. If a person has a hard time leaving food on the plate, this tool will help reduce calories without much effort. Use of colorful plates and utensils add to the enjoyment of mealtimes. Foods eaten in well-lit rooms are better than candlelight suppers. The darker the room, the easier it is to avoid seeing the amount of food being eaten.

It is important to have an environment that makes overeating impossible. Keeping favorite foods in the home where they are easily available is not a good idea. As long as the dieter knows that the favorite food is accessible, it will be a temptation. Treating oneself occasionally with a single serving of a favorite food is more appropriate and prevents over-obsession with the treat. If a person has an extreme craving, eating that food sparingly is much more desirable than binging on a whole container of cookies, ice cream, or chips because it is been banned as a "bad food".

Many dieters do not know how to listen to their body's hunger indicators. Learning how hunger feels allows them to make appropriate decisions on whether or not it is an appropriate time to eat. Sometimes the stomach will growl or feel cramped or "pinched". Some people feel lightheaded when hungry due to the drop in blood sugar. These are physical signs that it is time to eat. Eating when hungry enhances the flavor of food and makes meals more pleasurable.

Even though regular snacking between meals is not advisable, some may find that eating mini-meals that are more frequent 5-6 times daily helps to keep them from being overly hungry as opposed to the traditional three meals per day. Whichever plan works best for the individual is the way to success.

There are times when a person may believe they are hungry but in fact, they are thirsty. Drinking plenty of water and healthy fluids will keep the body hydrated and soften hunger pangs. This allows the dieter to get to the next meal without the temptation to over-indulge.

Finally, the importance of exercise cannot be overemphasized. Many dieters have found themselves overeating because of stressful situations. Exercise is an amazing stress reliever. Physical activity also serves as a very efficient appetite suppressant. When the temptation to overeat seems to be overwhelming, any activity that raises the cardiovascular rate will benefit the dieter's resolve. Exercise increases metabolism, which assists in the utilization of calories.

Proper planning is one of the best tools for preventing a relapse in overeating. Learning about the body's hunger signals, eating slowly, allowing occasional treats, and including exercise in the daily routine will all assist in getting the weight off and keeping it off for the long term.

ABOUT THE AUTHOR

Although Octavia Black has had her bouts with overeating, she's over it now because she understands what is behind it, which are emotions. Looking back in retrospect, it actually makes sense that that was where it was coming from. Emotions are so powerful and it can ruin you if you don't conquer it. But the key or secret is knowing how to do that.

She wishes that when she was going through it, there was a handy book available just like the one she has written because it really goes into the kind of detail required to help someone turn their emotions around in a healthy way that can only have a positive effect. Just like Octavia, everyone feels better when they look better and don't feel that they are too big or too fat from overeating. She wrote it in a way that would be easy for everyone to understand so that no one has an excuse for not at least trying to carry out some of the recommendations or suggestions - for their own good.

www.ingramcontent.com/pod-product-compliance
Lightning Source LLC
Chambersburg PA
CBHW070245290526
45789CB00004B/1776